CARD FILE ON
OCCUPATIONAL THERAPY ASSESSMENT IN MENTAL HEALTH

Barbara J. Hemphill, MS, OTR, FAOTA

SLACK INCORPORATED, 6900 GROVE ROAD, THOROFARE, NEW JERSEY 08086

SLACK International Book Distributors

In Europe, the Middle East and Africa.
  John Wiley & Sons Limited
  Baffins Lane
  Chichester, West Sussex P019 1UD
  England

In Canada:
  McAinsh and Company
  2760 Old Leslie Street
  Willowdale, Ontario M2K 2X5

In Australia and New Zealand:
  MacLennan & Petty Pty Limited
  P.O. Box 425
  Artarmon, N.S.W. 2064
  Australia

In Japan:
  Central Foreign Books Limited
  1-13 Jimbocho-Kanda
  Tokyo, Japan

In Asia and India:
  PG Publishing Pte Limited.
  36 West Coast Road, #02-02
  Singapore 0512

Foreign Translation Agent:
  John Scott & Company
  International Publishers' Agency
  417-A Pickering Road
  Phoenixville, PA 19460

Publisher: Harry C. Benson
Managing Editor: Lynn Borders
Editor: Stephanie Scanlon
Designer: Susan Hermansen
Production Coordinator: David Murphy

Printed in the United States of America

Library of Congress Catalog Card Number: 88-043592

ISBN: 1-556420-99-4

Published by: SLACK Incorporated
               6900 Grove Rd.
               Thorofare, NJ 08086

Last digit is print number: 10 9 8 7 6 5 4 3 2 1

CARD FILE ON OCCUPATIONAL THERAPY ASSESSMENT IN MENTAL HEALTH

INTRODUCTION

This card file of occupational therapy assessments in mental health is categorized into the four areas of human function. These areas of human function are described in Hemphill (1982), The Evaluative Process in Psychiatric Occupational Therapy, and Hemphill (1988), Mental Health Assessment in Occupational Therapy: An Integrative Approach to the Evaluative Process, Thorofare: Slack Incorporated. The reader is referred to these texts for explanation of each area of human function. Each area of human function is divided into sections marked by lettered tabs.

Two tables of contents are provided to assist the user in locating information about a specific assessment. The first provides names of assessments in alphabetical order. The second lists assessments according to each of the areas of human function. At the end of the card file is a bibliography of articles related to assessments used in occupational therapy mental health.

This material is to be used as a reference file to aid in the selection process. The lettered tabs and the tables of contents enhance easy access to assessments. Information about the assessment includes: the source from which the assessment can be obtained, the area of human function, the population, the necessary materials, the administration procedure, the research methodology and the scoring procedure.

In an attempt to provide information that is accurate and up to date, letters were sent to the authors of the assessments asking them to verify accuracy of the information. Having obtained information from the authors of the assessments, a literature review was undertaken to ascertain additional assessments. These assessments are included in this edition. No attempt is made to promote the value of the assessment or to promote any one theory or frame of reference.

ACKNOWLEDGEMENT

This author gratefully acknowledges Cheryl Linden, OTR for her countless hours as a research assistant. Her skills in research and data gathering enhanced the completion of this project. At the time of this writing Ms. Linden was a graduate student in occupational therapy at Western Michigan University.

Table of Contents
in Alphabetical Order

Assessment

Assessment

Table of Contents
According to Areas of Function

Assessment

I. Psychological (Section A)

II. Behavioral (Section B)

Assessment	Page

AZIMA BATTERY

Source: Hemphill, B. (Ed.). (1982). <u>The Evaluative Process in Psychiatric Occupational Therapy.</u> Thorofare: Charles B. Slack, Inc.

Theoretical Premise: Psychoanalytic, object relations.

Population: Adult, Neurosis, Personality Disorder, Psychosis.

Behaviors Assessed: Provides tactile, spatial, visual, auditory, olfactory stimulation. Evaluates reality contact, mood, level of functioning, quality of object relations, and ego control.

Research: Psychopharmacology changes. Therapy changes in individual and group therapy.

Administration: Projective test. The test is divided into the free association and inquiry phases. The client is asked to draw a person and then one of the opposite sex, to do something with clay, and to do a finger painting. Administered individually. Order of presentation is pencil, clay, finger painting.

A

Materials: Finger paints (yellow, red, green, blue, brown, and black). Container of water, clay, paper towels.

Area of Human Function: Psychological.

Normal Behavior Considered: No.

Interpretation: Behavioral Analysis, examination analysis.

Additional Sources:
Azima, H. (1961). Dynamic occupational therapy. <u>Disease of the Nervous System,</u> *22*(4).
Azima, H., & Azima, F. J. (1959). Outline of a dynamic theory of occupational therapy. <u>The American Journal of Occupational Therapy,</u> *13*(5).

B H BATTERY

Source: Hemphill, B. (1982). <u>Training Manual for the B H Battery</u>. Thorofare: Charles B. Slack, Inc.
Hemphill, B. (Ed.). (1982). <u>The Evaluative Process in Psychiatric Occupational Therapy</u>. Thorofare: Charles B. Slack, Inc.

Theoretical Premise: Analytical.

Population: Young adolescent, adult.

Behaviors Assessed: Follow directions, problem solve, frustration tolerance, abstraction, make decisions, organization, body concept, and feeling tone. Behaviors scored via rating scale.

Research: Inter-rater reliability.

A

Administration: Projective test. Procedure is clearly written in the training manual. It includes directions for setting up the activities. Procedure for recording the responses on the record form is described.

Materials: Mosaic tiling and finger painting. Equipment, materials, and environmental factors are included.

Area of Human Function: Psychological.

Normal Behavior Considered: Number 1 on the rating scale is considered normal response.

Interpretation: The training manual does not include interpretation. Interpretation of the B H Battery can be obtained from the discussion in the Evaluative Process. The meaning of scores needs researching.

CREATIVE CLAY TEST

Source: Hemphill, B. (Ed.). (1982). <u>The Evaluative Process in Psychiatric Occupational Therapy</u>. Thorofare, Charles B. Slack, Inc.

Theoretical Premise: Analytical; relationship between task structure and performance.

Population: Adult.

Behaviors Assessed: Performance on unstructured tasks.

Research: Case studies presented.

Administration: Projective test, scoring procedure is provided.

Materials: Clay, smooth board, time clock.

Area of Human Function: Psychological.

Normal Behavior Considered: Not discussed.

Interpretation: Guidelines are provided.

A

DIAGNOSTIC TEST BATTERY

Source: Androes, L., Dreyfus, E., & Bloesch, M. (1965). Diagnostic test battery for occupational therapy. The American Journal of Occupational Therapy, *19*(2).

Theoretical Premise: Analytical.

Population: Adult.

Behaviors Assessed: Not specific. Based on psychopathology inferences.

Research: None known.

Administration: Projective test. Task administered over a two- or four-hour period, often divided in two days. A series of questions is asked. Test contains five major parts.

A

Materials: Drawing, ceramics, painting, leatherwork and woodwork. Equipment and materials are thoroughly described.

Area of Human Function: Psychological.

Normal Behavior Considered: No.

Interpretation: Case studies described.

FIDLER BATTERY

Source: Fidler, G., & Fidler, J. (1963). <u>Occupational Therapy: A Communicative Process in Psychiatry</u>. New York: The Macmillan Co., page 104.

Theoretical Premise: Analytical, Azima.

Population: Not specified.

Behaviors Assessed: Concept of self, concept of others, ego organization, unconscious conflict, and communication.

Research: None.

Administration: Projective test. Procedure not discussed.

Materials: Projective material. Not specific.

Area of Human Function: Psychological.

Normal Behavior Considered: No.

Interpretation: Psychopathology inferences. Fidler discusses interpretation.

A

GOODMAN BATTERY

Source: Hemphill, B. (Ed.). (1982). <u>The Evaluative Process in Psychiatric Occupational Therapy</u>. Thorofare: Charles B. Slack, Inc.

Theoretical Premise: Analytical. Relationship between ego functioning and action. Goodman provides a literature review in mosaic tiling, drawing, and clay.

Population: Adolescent and adult; individuals with psychiatric disturbances. Used in inpatient and day care centers. Contraindications: heavily medicated patients, overly agitated or too disoriented clients.

Behaviors Assessed: Ego functioning. Four rating scales provided to rate organization, independence, self esteem: performance. Self esteem: verbal. Cognitive and affective: concept formation, organization, problem-solving ability, ego boundaries, with impulse control, reality testing and self-concept.

A

Research: None.

Administration: Projective test: Administered in one sitting. Standardized procedure is described in detail.

Materials: Mosaic tile, drawing, and clay. Described in detail.

Area of Human Function: Psychological.

Normal Behavior Considered: Rating scale is designed on a 7-point scale. Normal is scored 4.

Interpretation: Author provides guidelines. "Outline for Analysis of the Goodman Battery." Uses psychopathology inferences.

MAGAZINE PICTURE COLLAGE

Source: Hemphill, B. (Ed.). (1982). <u>The Evaluative Process in Psychiatric Occupational Therapy</u>. Thorofare: Charles B. Slack, Inc.

Theoretical Premise: Analytical, Azima, Buck and Provancher.

Population: Adult.

Behaviors Assessed: Personality organization: cognitive-perceptual function, quality of defenses, affect organization, object relations and sense of self.

Research: Inter-rater, construct validity, construct validity of the scoring system.

A

Administration: Projective test. Procedure is clearly described. A scoring system is used.

Materials: Glue, scissors, construction paper, and magazines.

Area of Human Function: Psychological.

Normal Behavior Considered: Not clear. Rating scale is not consistent.

Interpretation: More research needs to be done with rating scale. Author provides case studies.

Additional Sources:

Adelstein, L. A., & Nelson, D. L. (1985). Effects of sharing versus nonsharing on affective meaning in collage activities. Occupational Therapy in Mental Health, 5(2).

Buck, R., & Provancher, M. (1972). Magazine picture collage as an evaluation technique. The American Journal of Occupational Therapy, 26.

Carter, B. A., Nelson, D. L., & Duncombe, L. W. (1983). The effect of psychological type on mood and meaning of two collage activities. The American Journal of Occupational Therapy, *37*(10).

Lerner, C. (1979). The magazine picture collage: Its clinical use and validity as an assessment device. The American Journal of Occupational Therapy, *33*.

Lerner, C., & Ross, G. (1977). The magazine picture collage: Development of an objective scoring system. The American Journal of Occupational Therapy, *31*.

Sturgess, J. (1983). The magazine picture collage: A suitable basis for a pre-fieldwork teaching clinic. Occupational Therapy in Mental Health, *3*(1).

A

SHOEMYEN BATTERY

Source: Hemphill, B. (Ed.). (1982). <u>The Evaluative Process in Psychiatric Occupational Therapy</u>. Thorofare: Charles B. Slack, Inc.

Theoretical Premise: Analytical; Author claims an eclectic frame of reference.

Population: Adult.

Behaviors Assessed: Described in the administration procedure as self-confidence, artistic ability, suggestibility, concern for detail and design, perseveration, guardedness, problem-solving potential, dexterity, fine and gross motor skills. Forms are provided for recording responses.

Research: None; case studies are discussed. Based on psychopathological inferences.

A

Administration: Procedure is clearly written. It is written in terms of material and procedure, inherent qualities, and response variables.

Materials: Mosaic tile, finger painting, sculpture, and clay figure modeling.

Area of Human Function: Psychological.

Normal Behavior Considered: No.

Interpretation: Guidelines are provided. Based on psychopathological inferences.

Additional Sources:
Bendroth, S., & Southham, M. (1973). Objective evaluation of projective material. The American Journal of Occupational Therapy, *27*.

Shoemyen, C. (1970). Occupational therapy orientation and media. The American Journal of Occupational Therapy, *24*.

ACTIVITY CONFIGURATION

Source: Hemphill, B. (Ed.). (1982). <u>The Evaluative Process in Psychiatric Occupational Therapy</u>. Thorofare: Charles B. Slack, Inc., page 364.

Theoretical Premise: Occupational behavior and behavioral.

Population: Adult.

Behaviors Assessed: Balance of work, play/leisure, and self-maintenance activities.

Research: None.

Administration: Interview or self report.

Materials: Form and pencil.

B

Area of Human Function: Behavioral.

Normal Behavior Considered: Yes. A balance in work, play/leisure and self-maintenance is examined.

Interpretation: Inferred.

Additional Sources:
Denton, P. L. (1987). Psychiatric Occupational Therapy: A Workbook of Practical Skills. Boston: Little, Brown.

Hopkins, H., & Smith, H. (Eds.). (1973). Willard and Spackman's Occupational Therapy. New York: The Macmillan Co.

Mosey, A. (1973). Activities Therapy. New York: Raven Press.

ADOLESCENT FEMININE
OCCUPATIONAL BEHAVIOR DEVELOPMENT

Source: Pezzuti, L. (1979). An exploration of adolescent feminine and occupational behavior development. The American Journal of Occupational Therapy, *33*(2).

Theoretical Premise: Occupational behavior and behavioral.

Population: Female adolescent, ages 12-17.

Behaviors Assessed: Constructs: Sex-role identity and occupational choice.
Concepts: Peer relationships, independence, feminine social role, use of body, physique acceptance, occupational preparation.
A 3-point rating scale is used.

Research: None.

B

Administration: Self-evaluative tool. It is part of a battery including an interest checklist and a personal data sheet.

Materials: Rating form and a pencil.

Area of Human Function: Behavioral.

Normal Behavior Considered: Yes, Number 3 is rated normal. No overall score of normal behavior has been determined.

Interpretation: Based on inferences about occupational choice, cognitive development, awareness of values, interests, exposure to work and participation in play.

ADOLESCENT ROLE ASSESSMENT

Source: Hemphill, B. (Ed.). (1982). The Evaluative Process in Psychiatric Occupational Therapy. Thorofare: Charles B. Slack, Inc.

Theoretical Premise: Occupational choice.

Population: Adolescent, sex and age is not specified.

Behaviors Assessed: Family, school, and peer relationship. Occupational choice and work.

Research: Test-retest, validity studies on a small group of subjects.

Administration: Interview.

Materials: Rating form.

B

Area of Human Function: Behavioral.

Normal Behavior Considered: Plus scores suggest normal role behavior. Minus score suggests serious role behavior.

Interpretation: Score obtained from rating scale. Interpreted in terms of the behavior assessed.

Additional Sources:

Black, M. (1976). Adolescent role assessment. The American Journal of Occupational Therapy, *30*.

Denton, P. L. (1987). Psychiatric Occupational Therapy: A Workbook of Practical Skills. Boston: Little, Brown.

THE BARTH TIME CONSTRUCTION (BTC)

Source: Hemphill, B. (Ed.). (1988). <u>Mental Health Assessment in Occupational Therapy</u>. Thorofare: Slack, Inc.

Theoretical Premise: Behavioral. Person has to be functioning at Claudia Allen's Level 4. Activity configuration.

Population: Adolescent and adult populations. Alcohol/substance abuse.

Behaviors Assessed: How patient spends a week of time; used to build time management skills; can focus patients on the present; physical changes that require shifts in time use; planning as part of a rehabilitation treatment plan.

Research: Tested for inter-rater reliability. Content validity was established using Activity Analysis, Activity Configuration, Occupational History, and the Interest Checklist. See the BTC Manual.

B

Administration: In a group of three to six. Broken down into three parts: (1) summary format; (2) pre-cut strips of colors and a grid-like chart to complete. The resulting chart is a projective functioning self-image; and (3) C.O.T.E. scale.

Materials: Materials available in kit.

Area of Human Function: Behavioral.

Normal Behavior Considered: No.

Interpretation: How it was produced.
Gestalt of what was produced.
Content of what was produced.
Use of time with cognitive levels.

BAY AREA FUNCTIONAL PERFORMANCE EVALUATION (BaFPE)

Source: Hemphill, B. (Ed.). (1982). The Evaluative Process in Psychiatric Occupational Therapy. Thorofare: Charles B. Slack, Inc.

Theoretical Premise: Acquisitional and occupational behavior.

Population: Adult, psychiatric clients.

Behaviors Assessed: Task-Oriented Assessment: Paraphrasing, decision-making, organization of time, mastery and self-esteem, frustration tolerance, attention span, ability to abstract, mood disorder, task completion, and perceptual motor. The tasks yield information in four areas: cognition, performance, affect and qualitative signs, referral indicators.

B

Social Interaction Scale: Response to authority figures, verbal communication, independence/dependence, socially appropriate behavior, ability to work with peers, psychomotor behavior, participation in group or program activities.

The combined results of these two subtests are used as an indicator of patient's overall functional ability and provide information about patient cognition, affective, and motor functioning.

Research: Intra-rater, inter-rater, content validity, concurrent validity. The BaFPE correlates with the FLS and GAS. Construct validity was examined. Standardized on adult psychiatric inpatient population using 42 subjects for reliability and 62 for validity. The three subscales of the Wechsler Adult Intelligence Scale (WAIS) were administered in conjunction with the Task-Oriented Assessment (TOA). The picture completion, block design, and digit symbol correlated.

Administration: Procedure is standardized. An administration manual is provided. Preassessment Interview.

> Task-Oriented Assessment (TOA):
> Sorting Shells
> Bank Deposit Slip
> House Floor Plan
> Block Design
> Draw-A-Person

The Bank Deposit Slip is a more comprehensive money management task. Features such as grocery shopping and banking simulations have been added.

The House Floor Plan requires the subject to draw a well-structured plan, similar to a blueprint. The floor plan tasks contain more details to be memorized.

Perceptual-motor observations are scored via checklist.

Social Interaction Scale (SIS): Observation scale.

Takes 45-60 minutes to administer.

B

Materials: Materials are provided as part of the administration manual.

Area of Human Function: Behavioral.

Normal Behavior Considered: Yes. 4-point rating scale. 4 is the normal response.

Interpretation: The TOA is scored across 10 functional components and tallied. Subscores on (1) cognition, (2) performance, (3) affective. These scores are added to the scores from the SIS. Results give a profile of functional performance.

Additional Sources:

Bloomer, J. S., & Williams, S. (1982). The BaFPE Administration Manual (2nd printing). Palo Alto: Consulting Psychologist Press, Inc.

Bloomer, J. S., Williams, S., & Houston, D. (1980). The Bay Area Functional Performance Evaluation. Occupational Therapy in Mental Health, 1.

Denton, P. L. (1987). Psychiatric Occupational Therapy: A Workbook of Practical Skills. Boston: Little, Brown.

Thibeault, R., & Blackner, E. (1987). Validating a test of functional performance with psychiatric patients. The American Journal of Occupational Therapy, 41(8), 515.

B

INTEREST CHECKLIST

Source: Matsutsuyu, J. (1969). The interest checklist. <u>The American Journal of Occupational Therapy</u>, *23*(4).

Theoretical Premise: Occupational Behavior.

Population: Not specified.

Behaviors Assessed: Classify and describe interests of psychiatric patients by:
1) intensity of interest,
2) type of interest, and
3) ability to express personal preference.

Research: Test-retest.

B

Administration: Self-administered, check interest under the heading of casual, strong interest, and no interest. On reversed side the client is asked for a narrative report of: hobbies, pastimes, historical account of leisure time from grade school to the present.

Materials: Checklist.

Normal Behaviour Considered: None.

Area of Human Function: Behavioral.

Interpretation: Data is summarized into interest according to categories of manual skills, physical sports, social recreation, ADL and Cultural/Educational.

Additional Sources:

Denton, P. L. (1987). <u>Psychiatric Occupational Therapy: A Workbook of Practical Skills</u>. Boston: Little, Brown.

Hemphill, B. (1987). <u>Mental Health Assessments: An Integrative Approach to Occupational Therapy</u>. Thorofare: Slack, Inc.

Katz, N. (1988). Interest checklist: A factor analytical study. <u>Occupational Therapy in Mental Health</u>, *8*(1).

Rogers, et al. (1978). The interest checklist: An empirical assessment. <u>The American Journal of Occupational Therapy</u>, *32*(10).

B

LIFE STYLE PERFORMANCE PROFILE

Source: Hemphill, B. (Ed.). (1982). The Evaluative Process in Psychiatric Occupational Therapy. Thorofare: Charles B. Slack, Inc.

Theoretical Premise: Occupational Behavior and Behavioral.

Population: Adult.

Behaviors Assessed: Constructs:
    Care for and maintenance of self
    Intrinsic gratification
    Contribute to needs & welfare of others
  Concepts:
    Sensory/motor function
    Cognitive function
    Psychological function
    Dyadic and group skills

B

Research: None.

Administration: Interview, History of Performance, Occupational History.

Materials: Data-gathering form.

Area of Human Function: Behavioral.

Normal Behavior Considered: No.

Interpretation: Based on inferences.

OCCUPATIONAL CASE ANALYSIS (OCA)

Source: Kaplan, K. (1984). Short term assessment: The need and a response. <u>Occupational Therapy in Mental Health</u>, *4*(29).

Theoretical Premise: Human Occupation.

Population: Short-term, acutely ill psychiatric patients.

Behaviors Assessed: Personal causation, values/goals, interests, internalized roles, habit patterns, skills, output, physical environment, social environment, feedback.

Research: Inter-rater reliability, face and content validity.

Administration: Interview.

B

Materials: Form and pencil.

Area of Human Function: Behavioral.

Normal Behavior Considered: Results are rated on a scale of 1-5, with 5 being the most adaptive behavior.

Interpretation: Scoring protocol.

Additional Source:

Denton, P. L. (1987). Psychiatric Occupational Therapy: A Workbook of Practical Skills. Boston: Little, Brown, p. 73.

OCCUPATIONAL PERFORMANCE HISTORY INTERVIEW

Source: Hemphill, B. (Ed.). (1988). <u>Mental Health Assessment in Occupational Therapy</u>. Thorofare: Slack, Inc.

Theoretical Premise: Was formulated to be compatible with more than one frame of reference.

Population: To gather history of work, play, and self-care from psychosocially and/or physically disabled adolescents, adults and older persons.

B

Behaviors Assessed: Work, play and self-care. The questions cover 5 content areas:

1) Organization of daily living routines; how does the person spend their day
2) Life roles; what are the roles
3) Interests, values, and goals; how well does the person identify and act on roles
4) Perceptions of ability & responsibility; awareness of control over everyday life
5) Environment influences
   Life History Pattern

Research: Test-retest.

Administration: A recommended sequence and a format of questions is provided; the interviewer can add, delete, and adapt questions.

Materials: Paper and pencils.

Area of Human Function: Behavioral.

Normal Behavior Considered: 5-point rating scale.
Each content area consists of two items which are summed (past and present).
The five content areas are summed to obtain an overall score.
The higher the score, the more adapted.
Life History Pattern.

Interpretation: The higher the score, the more adapted.

Reference: Kielhofner, G., & Henry, A. (1988). Development and investigation of the occupational performance history interview. The American Journal of Occupational Therapy, *42*(8), 489.

B

THE OCCUPATIONAL FUNCTIONING TOOL (OFT)

Source: Watts, J. H., Kielhofner, G., Bauer, Gregory, & Valentine. (in press). The assessment of occupational functioning: Development of a screening instrument for use in long term care facilities. The American Journal of Occupational Therapy.

Theoretical Premise: Human Occupation.

Population: Institutionalized elderly.

Behaviors Assessed: Values, personal causation, interests, roles, habits, and skills.

Research: Test-retest reliability, inter-rater reliability, content validity. Concurrent validity with the Life Satisfaction Index-Z.

B

Administration: Administration protocol: interview.

Materials: Form, paper, and pencil.

Area of Human Function: Behavioral.

Normal Behavior Considered: Results rated on a scale of 1-5, with 1 as the most functional behavior.

Interpretation: Scoring protocol.

Additional Source:

Denton, P. L. (1987). Psychiatric Occupational Therapy: A Workbook of Practical Skills. Boston: Little, Brown, p. 73.

OCCUPATIONAL ROLE HISTORY

Source: Florey, L., & Michelman, S. (1982). Occupational role history: A screening tool for psychiatric occupational therapy. The American Journal of Occupational Therapy, *36*(5).

Theoretical Premise: Occupational Behavior. Based on the five assumptions identified by Moorhead. The assumptions basic to a life history of the occupational role:
1) There is a developmental progression in the acquisition of role skills throughout the life cycle. Experiences in earlier roles have direct impact on skills and habits required for future roles.
2) The family, school, peer group, and work setting help prepare and maintain an individual in his/her occupational role.

B

48

3) Critical components of skill acquisition are role models, method of role preparation, opportunities for role rehearsal, and areas of satisfaction or dissatisfaction.

4) Individuals are more vulnerable to negative effects of stress during periods of transition from one occupational role to another.

5) A qualitative balance between work and play activities is central to current function and preparation for future occupational roles.

Population: Adult.

Behaviors Assessed: To quickly identify and classify critical information in:

    1) Patterns of skills and achievement or patterns of dysfunction in occupational role.

    2) Balance in leisure activities and occupational role.

Research: A pilot study was conducted. No statistical procedure was conducted.

Administration: Semi-structured interview. The "Occupational Role Screening Interview" is used as a guide.

Materials: Question form.

Area of Human Function: Behavioral.

Normal Behavior Considered: No.

B

Interpretation: Categorized along two dimensions: Role status and balance.

> **Role Status:**
>
> > **Functional:** Pattern of skills and achievement were present, and good in past and current occupational role.
> >
> > **Temporarily impaired:** Occupational role skills were present in the past, but because they were interrupted, needing intervention.
> >
> > **Dysfunctional:** Sporadic patterns of skills in the past and current, needing intervention.
>
> **Balance:** Identified interests, hobbies, and activities he/she did on a consistent basis.

Additional Sources:

Denton, P. L. (1987). Psychiatric Occupational Therapy: A Workbook of Practical Skills. Boston: Little, Brown.

Moorhead, L. (1969). The occupational history. The American Journal of Occupational Therapy, 23.

PLAY SKILLS INVENTORY (PSI)

Source: Hurff, J. M. (1980). A play skills inventory: A competency monitoring tool for the 10 year old. The American Journal of Occupational Therapy, *34*(10), 651-656.

Theoretical Premise: Occupational Behavior/Occupational Choice.

Population: 8-12 year olds.

Behaviors Assessed: Gross deficit in sensory, motor, perception and intellectual behaviors.

Research: Piloted on 11 boys and 10 girls, aged 10.

Administration: Intent not to standardize. May use guidelines of the Competency Model.

Materials: Competency Model guidelines.

Area of Human Function: Behavioral.

Normal Behavior Considered: No.

Interpretation: Inferred.

THE ROLE ACTIVITY PERFORMANCE SCALE (RAPS)

Source: Good-Ellis, M., Fine, & Spencer. (1985). Developing a role activity performance scale. <u>The American Journal of Occupational Therapy</u>, *41*(4), 232.

Theoretical Premise: Occupational Behavior.

Population: Adult psychiatric patients: useful in the diagnostic, treatment, and discharge process. Will discriminate between schizophrenia and affective disorder.

Behaviors Assessed: Measures functional skills in 12 areas: work or work equivalent, education, home management, nuclear and extended family relationships, mate relationship, parental role, social relationships, leisure activities, self-management, health-care role, hygiene and appearance, and rehabilitation treatment settings.

B

Research: Some roles have concurrent validity with the Social Adjustment Scale-II, the Global Assessment Scale, and DSM III, Axis 5. Validity was tested in three ways: (a) review by experts, (b) tests of discrimination, (c) comparison with standardized measures.

Administration: Therapist can select among the 12 areas that are relevant and require evaluation. Administration protocol: Semi-structured interview; uses 12 subscales that represent a range of life roles.

Materials: Rating form and pencil.

Area of Human Function: Behavioral.

Normal Behavior Considered: Results scored from 1 to 6, with 1 being most functional.

Interpretation: Scoring protocol.

Additional Source:

Denton, P. L. (1987). <u>Psychiatric Occupational Therapy: A Workbook of Practical Skills</u>. Boston: Little, Brown, p. 73.

B

THE ROLE CHECKLIST

Source: Oakley, F., Kielhofner, G., Barris, R., & Reichler, D. K. (1986). The role checklist: Development and empirical assessment of reliability. The Occupational Therapy Journal of Research, 6(3), 57-161.

Theoretical Premise: Occupational Behavior (Role Theory). The concept of volition.

Population: Adolescent, adult, or geriatric population with physical or psychosocial dysfunction.

Behaviors Assessed: Present, past, future roles. Addresses four dimensions of roles: perceived incumbency, occupational role career, role balance, and role value.

B

Research: Content validity.
                Test-retest reliability.

Administration: Two parts: Part 1 assesses along a temporal continuum. Part 2 measures the degree to which the individual values each role.

Materials: Written inventory.

Area of Human Function: Behavioral.

Normal Behavior Considered: Not addressed.

Interpretation: In development, normative data needed.

Part 1:

Past refers to any time up to the immediately preceding week.

Present includes the day the checklist is completed, as well as the previous seven days.

Future is any time from tomorrow onward.

Part 2:

Individuals are instructed to check the column that best describes the value they attributed to each role even if they have not performed or do not anticipate performing the role.

B

BASIC LIVING SKILLS (CEBLS)

Source: Casanova, J., & Ferber, J. (1976). Comprehensive evaluation of basic living skills. The American Journal of Occupational Therapy, *30*(2).

Theoretical Premise: Acquisition of basic living skills.

Population: Chronic patients. Contraindicated for acute clients, crisis intervention and short-term treatment facilities.

Behaviors Assessed: Personal care and hygiene: Ability to clothe, wash, and self-groom and to perform light housekeeping tasks.

Practical evaluation: Plans and prepares a meal, uses public transportation and the telephone.

Written evaluation: Ability to read, ability to write, understand time, solve math problems and manage money.

C

Research: None.

Administration: Nursing staff: Observation of Care and Hygiene Checklist.
O.T. staff: Observation of Practical Evaluation. Takes as long as eight hours to administer. A rating scale is used to guide observations.

Materials: Checklist.

Area of Human Function: Learning.

Normal Behavior Considered: Behaviors are rated on a 1-4 continuum; 4 is the highest function.

Interpretation: Score is added and multiplied by 4.

BASIC LIVING SKILLS BATTERY (BLSB)

Source: Skolaski-Pellitteri, T., & Chapman-Broekema, M. <u>The basic living skills battery: A tool for assessing adjustment to community living</u>. Unpublished manuscript.

Theoretical Premise: Adjustment to community living for adult psychiatric clients.

Population: Adult ages 18-65. Prolonged periods of hospitalization.

Behaviors Assessed: Living arrangements, employment, money management, transportation, communication, recreation, interpersonal relationships, personal care and hygiene, sexual knowledge, personal feelings scale, medical care, and impression of mental status.

C

Research: None.

Administration: Questionnaire. Can be administered in one sitting. Client completes Personal Data Sheet. Personal care and hygiene by observation.

Materials: Questionnaire, Personal Data Sheet.

Area of Human Function: Learning.

Normal Behavior Considered: No.

Interpretation: Level of functioning is inferred.

BEHAVIOR RATING SCALE

Source: Wolff, R. (1961). A behavior rating scale. <u>The American Journal of Occupational Therapy</u>, *15*(1).

Theoretical Premise: Evaluation of patient progress, and effectiveness of therapies, and determination of readiness to leave hospital. Based on the MFS Rehabilitation Evaluation Scale.

Population: Adult, aid in observation of patients in state mental hospitals.

Behaviors Assessed: Response to work, activity or task: Interest, follow through, follow directions, work with others, quality and quantity of work.
Response to people: attitude, hostility, verbalization.
General observation: independence/dependence.

C

Research: Inter-rater studies, face validity, reliability over time, content validity, meaning of scores was examined.

Administration: Observation rating scale from normal to abnormal.

Materials: MFS Rehabilitation Rating Scale.

Area of Human Function: Learning.

Normal Behavior Considered: Yes.

Interpretation: Score was examined for meaning. No score was reported.

THE COGNITIVE ADAPTIVE SKILLS EVALUATION (CASE)

Source: Masagatani, G. N., Nielson, C. S., & Ranslow, E. K. (1980). The cognitive adaptive skills evaluation. Occupational Therapy in Mental Health, *1*(2), 43-44.

Theoretical Premise: Piaget, Mosey, Singer: Intended to survey functional skills. Not a predictor of future behavior.

Population: Psychiatric patients.

Behaviors Assessed: Individual's cognitive process while engaged in the performance of a task.

Research: Field tested on non-patients and then on patients for one year; reliability and validity studies done; still being researched. No quantitative scores reported.

Administration: Patient is asked to perform a paper and pencil task and to respond to interview questions related to the task. After responding to interview questions, the person repeats the task and responds to a second set of interview questions related to both tasks.

Materials: Paper, pencil, form.

Area of Human Function: Learning.

Normal Behavior Considered: Not reported.

Interpretation: Results summarized and analyzed according to predetermined behavioral criteria. There are no quantitative scores reported about this evaluation.

COMPREHENSIVE OCCUPATIONAL THERAPY EVALUATION (COTE)

Source: Hemphill, B. (Ed.). (1982). The Evaluative Process in Psychiatric Occupational Therapy. Thorofare: Charles B. Slack, Inc.

Theoretical Premise: Eclectic.

Population: Adult, acute psychiatric setting.

Behaviors Assessed: General behavior: Appearance, nonproductive behavior, activity level, expression, responsibility, punctuality, reality orientation.
Interpersonal relationships: Independence, self-assertion, sociability, ability to get attention, response from others.

C

Task performance: Engagement, concentration or attention span, coordination, following directions, activity neatness, attention to detail, problem solving, organization of tasks, initial learning, interest, decision-making, and frustration tolerance.

Research: Inter-rater reliability. Validity was examined by comparing 56 charts of discharged patients.

Administration: Observation. A rating scale is provided. Rating is from 0 to 4. Scores are summed.

Materials: Rating Scale. Activity is chosen by the therapist. Most activity can be used.

Area of Human Function: Learning.

Normal Behavior Considered: Score is added. Score of less than 10 indicates readiness for discharge.

Interpretation: Based on scores obtained. Inferred from observation of behavior during activity.

Additional Sources:

Brayman, S., et al. (1976). Comprehensive occupational therapy evaluation scale. The American Journal of Occupational Therapy, *30*(2).

Denton, P. L. (1987). Psychiatric Occupational Therapy: A Workbook of Practical Skills. Boston: Little, Brown, P. 80.

C

FORM TO EVALUATE WORK BEHAVIORS

Source: Ayres, A. J. (1954). A form used to evaluate the work behavior of patients. The American Journal of Occupational Therapy, 8(2).

Theoretical Premise: Physical capacity of the patient to engage in work activities, and on-the-spot evaluation of work behavior.

Population: Adult.

Behaviors Assessed: Work behaviors.

Research: None; valid only for work behaviors while receiving occupational therapy.

C

Administration: Observation while in work behavior. Activity is not specified.

Materials: Rating scale.

Area of Human Function: Learning.

Normal Behavior Considered: Questions are checked according to the percentage of time. The number of checks in each column is multiplied by the number indicated at the bottom of the column.

Interpretation: Inferred from the rating scale.

THE INDEPENDENT LIVING SKILLS EVALUATION

Source: Johnson, T. P., Vinnicombe, B. J., & Merrill, G. W. (1980). The independent living skills evaluation. Occupational Therapy in Mental Health, *1*(2), 5-18.

Theoretical Premise: Community living skills.

Population: Chronic mentally disabled persons living in community-based satellite apartment programs.

Behaviors Assessed: Performance in money management, shopping and consumer education, meal preparation and storage, house cleaning and maintenance, personal hygiene and clothing maintenance, medication management and health care, community resources and transportation, communication and interpersonal relations, problem solving and decision making, vocational and personal growth.

Evaluates skills necessary for independent community living in the areas of household maintenance, personal and health care, community resources, communication, and problem solving, and vocational and personal growth.

Research: Has been used as an experimental evaluation tool with a small client sample.

Administration: Therapist report and self-report by client; 2½ hour administration time. Standardized procedure.

Materials: Score sheet and pencil and description of the ten major areas to be evaluated.

Area of Human Function: Learning.

Normal Behavior Considered: Scale graded on a 1-4 continuum, 4 describing the optimal level of functioning.

Interpretation: Behavioral descriptions used for scoring each category are used in setting objectives. An example of using behavioral descriptions for scoring is:

Money Management—Banking transactions

4 - Can accurately describe the procedures involved in using checking and savings accounts, getting a money order, cashing a check, and opening a bank account. Demonstrates the ability to balance a checkbook accurately.

3 - Can accurately describe the procedure involved in using a savings account, getting a money order, cashing a check and opening bank accounts. Unable to accurately register checks and balance a checkbook and/or frequently bounces checks.

C

2 - Can accurately describe the procedures involved in getting a money order and cashing a check. Unable to accurately use a savings or checking account.

1 - Unable to independently purchase a money order, cash a check, or accurately use a savings or checking account.

Additional Source:

Marks, R. (1980). Validating the I.L.S.E. Occupational Therapy in Mental Health, *1*(2), 19-20.

To obtain the complete I.L.S.E.:

Toni Johnson
Independent Living Project
291 North Tenth Street
San Jose, CA 95112
(408) 279-1975

THE JACOBS PREVOCATIONAL SKILLS ASSESSMENT (JPSA)

Source: Jacobs, K. (1985). <u>Occupational Therapy: Work-related Programs and Assessments</u>. Boston: Little, Brown.

Theoretical Premise: Occupational choice.

Population: Learning disabled adolescent.

Behaviors Assessed: 15 tasks designed to assess performance in specific work-related skill areas.

Research: None.

Administration: Task performance. Standardized procedure.

C

Materials: Tasks are: Quality control, filing, carpentry assembly, classification, office work, use of a telephone directory, factory work, environmental mobility, money concepts, functional banking, time concepts, work attitude, body scheme, leather assembly and food preparation. Supplies are listed in resource.

Area of Human Function: Learning.

Normal Behavior Considered: Completion of tasks.

Interpretation: Scoring protocol: results are summarized. Resource provides case studies.

KOHLMAN EVALUATION OF LIVING SKILLS (KELS)

Source: McGourty, L. (1979). <u>Kohlman evaluation of living skills</u>. Unpublished manuscript.

Theoretical Premise: Person's ability to function in basic living skills.

Population: Inpatient psychiatric treatment setting. Appropriate for mentally retarded, organic brain syndrome, geriatric and brain injured.

Behaviors Assessed: Self-care, safety and health, money management, transportation and telephone, work and leisure.

Research: Six studies completed—validity and reliability studies.

Administration: Task performance and interview. Procedure is clearly written for each area assessed. Manual is provided.

Materials: Material is provided via manual. Manual can be obtained from: KELS Research, Box 33503, Seattle, WA 98133.

Area of Human Function: Learning.

Normal Behavior Considered: Behaviors are assessed on independence; needs assistance continuum.

Interpretation: A final score is computed. Each section marked "needs assistance" is scored 1 point. Work and leisure is scored ½ point. A total score of 5½ or less indicates capable of independent living.

Additional Source:

Denton, P. L. (1987). Psychiatric Occupational Therapy: A Workbook of Practical Skills. Boston: Little, Brown.

MILWAUKEE EVALUATION OF DAILY LIVING SKILLS

Source: Hemphill, B. (Ed.). (1988). Mental Health Assessment in Occupational Therapy. Thorofare: Slack, Inc.

Theoretical Premise: Behavioral performance of functional living skills.

Population: Chronically mentally ill.

Behaviors Assessed: Assessment of behaviors/skills needed for adequate functioning in client's anticipated living situation. Basic communication skills, dressing, eating, maintenance of clothing, medicine management, personal care, and hygiene, toileting, brushing teeth, denture care, bathing, use of make-up, shaving, nail care, hair care, eyeglass care, personal health care, safety in community, safety in home, time awareness, use of money, use of telephone, use of transportation.

Research: Underway—inter-rater reliability.

Administration: 21 subtests. Screening form (Appendix D) Serves as a quick reference to which skill areas need to be evaluated.

Materials: Normal consumer products.

Area of Human Function: Learning.

Normal Behavior Considered: Yes. The reporting form indicates the skill of the performance needed. There is no cumulative score.

Additional Sources:

Leonardelli, C. (1986). The process of developing a quantifiable evaluation of daily living skills in psychiatry. Occupational Therapy in Mental Health, 6(4), 17.

Leonardelli, C. (1988). The Milwaukee Evaluation of Daily Living Skills. Thorofare: Slack, Inc.

PARACHEK GERIATRIC RATING SCALE

Source: Parachek, J., & King, L. J. (1982). <u>Parachek Geriatric Rating Scale</u>. Phoenix: Center for Neurodevelopmental Studies, Inc.

Theoretical Premise: A short ADL screening tool that categorizes patients into specific therapeutic regimes.

Population: Hospitalized geriatric patients.

Behaviors Assessed: Behavior is measured on a 5-point rating scale.
Physical Condition: Ambulation, eyesight, hearing.
General Self-care: Toilet habits, eating, hygiene, and grooming.
Social Behaviors: Helps with work on ward, individual responses, group activities.

C

Research: Standardized for age 65 and older.
Standardized on 150 patients.
Measured changes in treatment groups.
Treatment groups are described in the manual.

Administration: A quick initial screening tool. The procedure is to observe the present condition of the patient.

Materials: Rating form and record form.

Area of Human Function: Learning.

Normal Behavior Considered: Yes. Number 5 is considered normal behavior.

Interpretation: A total score is obtained and recorded on the record form to aid visual progress. The total score is used to guide the therapist in deciding which treatment group the patient is placed. Patients are grouped according to their functional level. The manual gives treatment procedures for each group.

Additional Source:

Miller, E. R., Parachek, J. R. (1974). Validation and standardization of a goal-oriented, qiuck-screening geriatric scale. Journal of the American Geriatrics Society, *22*(6).

Manual can be obtained from:
Center for Neurodevelopmental Studies, Inc.
8430 North 39th Avenue, North Suite
Phoenix, AZ 85051

PRE-VOCATIONAL ASSESSMENT OF PSYCHIATRIC PATIENTS

Source: Ethridge, D. (1968). Pre-vocational assessment of rehabilitation potential of psychiatric patients. The American Journal of Occupational Therapy, *12*(3).

Theoretical Premise: Vocational potential of patients considered for rehabilitation.

Population: Adult psychiatric patients.

Behaviors Assessed: Work skills, habits and tolerance, socialization, attitude toward others, personality characteristics, and general observation.

Research: Internal consistency. Each of the four sections were related to successful rehabilitation.

C

Administration: Observation. Items are arranged on a 4-point rating scale from very poor to excellent.

Materials: Rating scale.

Area of Human Function: Learning.

Normal Behavior Considered: There are 20 items. A score of 60 or above indicates good work adjustment.

Interpretation: Based on a score of 60.

Additional Source:

Distefano, M. K., & Pryer, M. W. (1970). Vocational evaluation and successful placement of psychiatric clients in a vocational rehabilitation program. The American Journal of Occupational Therapy, 24(3).

THE SCORABLE SELF-CARE EVALUATION (SSCE)

Source: Peters, M., & Clark, N. (1984). The Scorable Self-Care Evaluation. Thorofare: Charles B. Slack, Inc.

Theoretical Premise: Acquisitional.

Population: Psychosocially dysfunctional.

Behaviors Assessed: Personal care: Appearance, orientation, hygiene, communications, and first aid.
Housekeeping: Food selection, house chores, safety, laundry.
Work and leisure: Leisure activity, transportation, job seeking.
Financial management: Making correct change, checking, bill paying, budgeting, source of income.

C

Research: Test reliability, test-retest, inter-rater, normative data.

Administration: Interview and task performance. The administration manual provides instructions for each subtask.

Materials: Scorable Self Care Scoring Form, Orientation Form, Food Menu Form, Budget Form, Check Form, Laundry Form. Forms included with manual. Permission to copy forms.

Area of Human Function: Learning.

Normal Behavior Considered: The SSCE has a negative scoring system. Scores are given for inability to perform task. The smaller the total score, the more functional the individual. Normative data includes 67 adults, ages 13-69.

Interpretation: Normative data provided.

Additional Source:

Denton, P. L. (1987). <u>Psychiatric Occupational Therapy: A Workbook of Practical Skills</u>. Boston: Little, Brown.

ADULT PSYCHIATRIC SENSORY-INTEGRATIVE EVALUATION (SBC)

Source: Hemphill, B. (Ed.). (1982). <u>The Evaluative Process in Psychiatric Occupational Therapy</u>. Thorofare: Charles B. Slack, Inc.

Theoretical Premise: There are perceptual and motor disturbances in psychiatric illness— schizophrenia.

Population: Adult.

Behaviors Assessed: <u>Sensory</u> and <u>motor responses</u> including reflex integration, fine and motor skills and neurologic soft signs. Dominance, posture, neck rotation, gait, hand observation, grip strength, fine-motor control, diadochokineses, finger-thumb opposition, visual pursuits, bilateral coordination, crossing the midline, stability, classical Romberg, overflow movements, neck righting, rolling, ATNR, STNR, tonic labyrinthine, protective extension, seated equilibrium, body image, <u>abnormal movements</u>, self-reported childhood history.

D

Research: Inter-rater, validity studies, construct validity supported. Internal consistency. Recent research demonstrates (1) that the SBC is sensitive to sensory integrative dysfunction; (2) sensorimotor responsiveness and physical performance, on the average, decline with increasing age; (3) a psychiatric group will obtain higher scores than a comparison group; (4) antipsychotic medication was associated with more disordered functioning on the physical assessment and abnormal movements subscales.

Administration: Procedure is standardized: Abnormal movement subscale, childhood history subscale, physical assessment subscale.

Materials: A work sheet and equipment list are provided in the manual. Some equipment needed: paper tube, cardboard, metal key ring, pencil, paper, rubber ball, goniometer, jamar dynamometer, tapping board, stop watch, pen light, blackboard, chalk, masking tape, mat and safety belt.

Area of Human Function: Biological.

Normal Behavior Considered: 0 on the rating scale is considered normal.

Interpretation: Objective observations. Norms on adult population - 113 psch - 31 norms.

Additional Sources:

Schroeder, C., Block, M., Trottier, E., & Stowell, M. (1981). Adult Psychiatric Sensory Integration Evaluation. Kailua: Carolyn Schroeder Consultant and Publisher.

Schroeder, C., & Herbert, A. (1981). Adult Psychiatric Sensory Integration Treatment Manual. Kailua: Carolyn Schroeder Consultant and Publisher.

Wong, G., & Schroeder, C. (1981). For Seniors Only: Health Care Maintenance. Kailua: Carolyn Schroeder Consultant and Publisher.

D

THE ROUTINE TASK HISTORY (RTH)

Source: Allen, C. K. (1985). <u>Occupational Therapy for Psychiatric Diseases: Measurement and Management of Cognitive Disabilities</u>. Boston: Little, Brown.

Theoretical Premise: Cognitive disabilities.

Population: Acutely ill adult psychiatric patients.

Behaviors Assessed: Living situation, social support, self-care responsibilities, work history, educational history, interests, recent typical day, past hospitalizations, and patient's assessment of his/her assets, limitations, and goals.

Administration: Administration protocol: Interview; client needs to be at level 3 or 4. Questions: Living situation, social support, self-care, work, educational, interest, typical day.

D

Materials: Form and pencil.

Area of Human Function: Biological.

Normal Behavior Considered: Level 6; DSM III - Axis 5.

Interpretation: Scoring protocol: according to the six levels of cognition.

Additional Source:

Denton, P. L. (1987). Psychiatric Occupational Therapy: A Workbook of Practical Skills. Boston: Little, Brown, p. 73.

THE WORK PERFORMANCE INVENTORY

Source: Allen, C. K. (1985). <u>Occupational Therapy for Psychiatric Diseases: Measurement and Management of Cognitive Disabilities</u>. Boston: Little, Brown.

Theoretical Premise: Cognitive levels.

Population: Psychiatric patients in workshop environment.

Behaviors Assessed: Work habits, work relationships, motor skills, perceptions and emotions affecting work performance, cognitive levels, self-regulation.

D

Research: None found.

Administration: Observation.

Materials: Form and pencil.

Area of Human Function: Biological.

Normal Behavior Considered: Level 6/3 on rating scale.

Interpretation: According to cognitive levels.

REFERENCE LIST

Auerbuch, S., & Katz, N. (1988). Assessment of perceptual cognitive performance: Comparison of psychiatric and brain injured adult patients. Occupational Therapy in Mental Health, 8(1).

Bell, C. H., Kavanaugh, M. M., Ridout, K. C., & Gainer, F. E. (1986). A strategy for assessing occupational behavior: Part II. An inter-rater reliability study. Occupational Therapy in Mental Health, 6(3), 1-17.

Bocks, T., Gordon, H., & Brozost, B. A. (1981). Individualized psychosocial assessment of chronic psychiatric patients in a day treatment setting. Mental Health Special Interest Section Newsletter, 4(3), 90-92.

Clark, J. R., Koch, B. A., & Nichols, R. C. (1965). A factor analytically derived scale for rating psychiatric patients in occupational therapy: Part 1. Development. The American Journal of Occupational Therapy, 19(1), 14-17.

Coster, W. (1979). Assessing an assessment tool. <u>Developmental Disabilities Special Interest Section Newsletter,</u> *2*(3).

Culp, R. E., Packard, V. N., & Humphry, R. (1980). Sensorimotor versus cognitive-perceptual training effects on the body concept of preschoolers. <u>The American Journal of Occupational Therapy,</u> *34*(4), 259-262.

Dip, C. L. (1986). The process of goal setting using goal attainment scaling in a therapeutic community. <u>Occupational Therapy in Mental Health,</u> *6*(3), 19-30.

Esenther, S. (1978). A response to: Use of the goal attainment scale in the treatment and ongoing evaluation of neurologically handicapped children. <u>The American Journal of Occupational Therapy,</u> *32*(8), 511.

Heine, D., & Steiner, M. (1986). Standardized paintings as a proposed adjunct instrument for longitudinal monitoring of mood states: A preliminary note. <u>Occupational Therapy in Mental Health,</u> *6*(3), 31-37.

Jacobson, A., & Adamson, J. D. (1973). Relationships of picture content and patient's age and diagnosis to color choice. The American Journal of Occupational Therapy, 27(1), 40-43.

Kannegieter, R. B. (1986). The development of the environmental assessment scale. Occupational Therapy in Mental Health, 6(3), 67-83.

Kaplan, K. (1984). Short-term assessment: The need and a response. Occupational Therapy in Mental Health, 4(3), 29-45.

Lewinsohn, P. M., & Clark, J. R. (1965). A factor analytically derived scale for rating psychiatric patients in occupational therapy: Part II. Concurrent validity. The American Journal of Occupational Therapy, 19(2), 72-75.

Llorens, L. A. (1967). Projective technique in occupational therapy. The American Journal of Occupational Therapy, 21(4), 226-229.

Marvin, P. (1979). Assessment of the pre-vocational/vocational client. Developmental Disabilities Special Interest Section Newsletter, 2(4), 36.

Platzer, W. S. (1976). Effect of perceptual motor training on gross-motor skill and self-concept of young children. The American Journal of Occupational Therapy, 30(7), 422-428.

Rider, B. A. (1978). Sensorimotor treatment of chronic schizophrenics. The American Journal of Occupational Therapy, 32(7), 451-455.

Snow, T. (1979). The multidimensional functional assessment questionnaire. Gerontology Special Interest Section Newsletter, 2(3), 71.

Snow, T. (1983). Assessing mental status. Gerontology Special Interest Section Newsletter, 6(1), 52-53.

Snow, T. (1983). Assessing self-care status. Gerontology Special Interest Section Newsletter, 6(2), 51-52.

Stauffer, D. L. (1986). Predicting successful employment in the community for people with a history of chronic mental illness. Occupational Therapy in Mental Health, 6(2), 31-49.